Your Gum Graft

What to Expect & How to Make it Easy!

(Including 7 Healthy Recipes)

Susan G. Clark

"This book will be helpful and informative for patients receiving a gum graft. *Your Gum Graft: What to Expect & How to Make it Easy!* is a great idea."

— Antonio Moretti, DDS, MS, Associate Professor and Graduate Program Director, Department of Periodontology, UNC School of Dentistry

Acknowledgements

To Antonio Moretti, DDS, MS, Associate Professor and Graduate Program Director, Department of Periodontology, UNC School of Dentistry, for his invaluable input.

To Alison McGuire, DMD, 2014 Graduate, Department of Periodontology, UNC School of Dentistry, for her superior care and expertise during two gum grafts surgeries and a dental implant.

To my dear Raphael, for his incredible support and encouragement.

To the two funny felines, for their devotion and constant companionship.

Your Gum Graft: What to Expect & How to Make it Easy! is available at http://www.Amazon.com/author/susangclark.

Susan G. Clark, an author in Raleigh, North Carolina, has been the recipient of three gum grafts within the span of eighteen months. Susan professes, "It's really much easier than you think!"

Subscribe to Susan's e-mail at http://www.susangclark.com to receive her free assessment for determining if you are stuck in humdrum plus tips to help you transition from humdrum to holy crap! You will also receive occasional notices about new blog posts, books, and instructional videos.

Contents

Getting the Gum Graft News

So you finally agreed to see a specialist about your gums. Good for you!

You've probably put this off for a while, hoping your little problem would go away. But it didn't. After your regular dentist repeatedly pointed out that your little problem wouldn't be going away without some big help from a specialist, you began to pay attention. And now that specialist—the periodontist you agreed to visit just to talk—tells you that you need a gum graft. Maybe two.

And I'd be willing to bet that you took the gum graft news reasonably well, right up to the part where the periodontist described the procedure. Then it began to sound a little scary. Like something you might want to skip entirely.

Well, as off-putting as the procedure might sound, a gum graft experience can be a breeze. I know, because I've had three.

" I will be the first to admit that I have never enjoyed being on the receiving end of dental work. "

The First of My Three Gum Grafts

Although early in my career I was briefly employed as a dental receptionist and hygienist's assistant, I will be the first to admit that I have never enjoyed being on the receiving end of dental work. But we do what we have to do, don't we.

So I made an appointment with a periodontist.

The periodontist echoed what my dentist had told me. My gums had receded to the extent that the roots of many of my lower teeth were partially exposed. As a result, I was experiencing sensitivity to hot and cold, had grown increasingly unhappy with the appearance of my teeth, and, despite taking great care to brush correctly, watched as the gum recession only got worse.

According to the American Academy of Periodontology, "A gum graft can reduce further recession and bone loss. In some cases, it can cover exposed roots to protect them from decay. This may reduce tooth sensitivity and improve esthetics of your smile."

While the periodontist described my first graft—a Free Gingival Graft, which would require taking a strip of skin from the roof of my mouth, placing it over four (not one, not two; four!) of my practically exposed roots, and stitching that tissue securely in place—I silently calculated how much longer I might continue to put off the procedure. But I couldn't keep putting it off. It had to be done.

The periodontist suggested performing the first graft and a second graft on the same day, but because of annual insurance limits, I chose to schedule only the first graft, and it would need to be completed before the end of the year.

I chose a date and discussed my sedation options and payment arrangements. My head was buzzing when I headed out the door with a folder full of instructions, a signed agreement, and some prescriptions to have filled. The last time I'd felt so overwhelmed was after several hours at an auto dealership buying a car. Both present an incredibly stressful situation to the customer. The patient. Me. And now, you.

On the designated gum graft day, I had a friend drive me to my appointment. Before leaving home I swallowed three 2 mg diazepam tablets and, once I was settled in the chair, welcomed the nitrous oxide. Then I plugged the earbuds into my iPod, selected a favorite long-playing album, and closed my eyes. Let the party begin!

Before I knew it, the procedure was over. My part had been easy—the superb drugs that periodontists have available these days made it completely painless.

After graft one, I was sent home with a removable plastic shield protecting the roof of my mouth and some flexible gummy stuff protecting the new graft.

I had been given printed guidelines to follow for the next two to three weeks, instructing me to begin with a soft diet, avoid eating anything hard or crunchy, and avoid exercise or exertion for at least 24 hours.

To control swelling, it was recommended that I apply an ice pack every 10 minutes for the first four hours and sleep with my head elevated the first night. That I knew I could handle.

In the spirit of full disclosure, a little bleeding is normal the first day, but I was informed that it is easily controlled by gently applying pressure with either moist gauze or a tea bag.

And I was strictly instructed not to smoke, spit, or drink from a straw for the first 48 hours, nor disturb the graft by tugging on my lip "to check things out." I was also directed to avoid brushing or flossing the grafted area until the healing could be assessed at my next visit to the periodontist's office.

Regarding pain, I've heard from more than one expert in the medical community that it is far more effective to prevent pain than to stop pain once it has started. In my case, I was instructed to alternate acetaminophen and ibuprofen every six to eight hours to prevent discomfort. It worked for me. If you follow the pain management schedule recommended by your periodontist, you should be comfortable.

With prescriptions for a bottle of mouth rinse, which I wasn't to use until 24 hours had passed, and a five-day supply of anti-inflammatory meds, I was prepared. For what, I wasn't sure. Would I be able to eat? Drink? What about sleep? I know that if I don't get eight good hours of sleep every night, I don't function!

At the one-week follow-up appointment, my periodontist asked me about the days since my procedure. I shrugged and said it had been surprisingly easy. While it hadn't exactly been a normal week—I hadn't yet eaten anything that required chewing—overall, I'd felt great!

My Second Gum Graft

Eleven months later, when the opportunity arose to get the second gum graft, I jumped at it. I'd become unhappy with how my front teeth looked in photos. So I'm a little vain. Isn't everyone?

The second graft, a Soft Tissue Allograft, using tissue from a human donor instead of my own tissue, was even easier than the first.

During my appointment, I kept my finger on the volume control of my iPod to distract me from the activity and any conversation between the periodontist and her assistant that I didn't want to hear. As with the first graft, there wasn't any discomfort. However, take my word for it when I say you really will not want to think too much about what is going on. Trust that your periodontist knows what he or she is doing, turn up the volume, and just let him or her do the job.

Toward the end of the procedure, I overheard the periodontist begin to describe the suturing technique—subpapillary continuous sling sutures, which I later learned is a method that combines two types of graft sutures into a single continuous sling that goes between and around the teeth. Because I've always had a fascination with knots, first as a girl scout and then as a sailboat owner, I turned down my iPod to listen.

I was so impressed with the results that, at my follow-up appointment, I complimented my periodontist on her handiwork and requested a copy of the photographs. Aren't these sutures amazing!

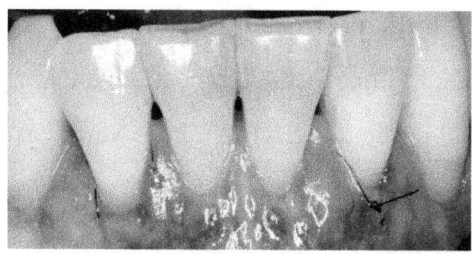

The fancy sutures: front view.

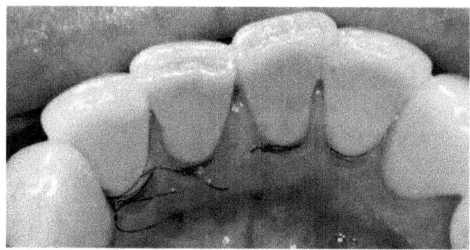

The fancy sutures: inside view.

Afterward, I headed home with prescriptions for another bottle of mouth rinse and a seven-day supply of amoxicillin and a plan for alternating doses of acetaminophen and ibuprofen. I didn't need the prescription pain meds and, four days later, I only occasionally needed any ibuprofen.

The inability to bite into food with my front teeth was inconvenient, but I adapted. It did slow me down a bit, but most of us could stand to eat a little more leisurely, right?

Two Kitchen Items You Will Need

First, get yourself a thin-rimmed white wine glass. It will make those first mealtimes so much easier. There is something about the shape of a white wine glass with a thin rim that delivers liquid nourishment—serious nourishment—to the back of the tongue incredibly efficiently. If you also enjoy a little wine with your dinner, you will need two glasses.

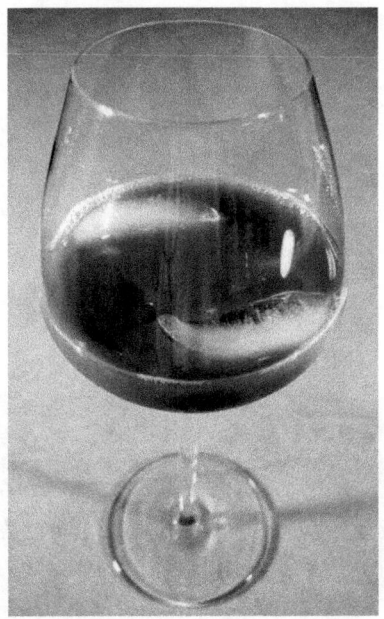

Thin-rimmed glass of iced coffee.

You will use the glass daily—in the mornings for fruit and yogurt smoothies, iced coffee or tea, and at dinner for pureed, chilled soup.

Second, after you've healed a bit and progressed beyond drinking your meals, you'll appreciate having a couple of small, narrow spoons available. I can't count the number of times I had to wash my single narrow iced tea spoon during the weeks following my gum grafts. I purchased mine from one of the large kitchen stores.

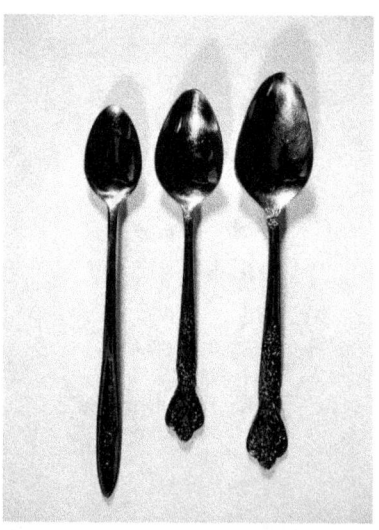

Iced tea spoon (left), and standard flatware teaspoon (middle), and tablespoon (right).

Also, if you don't have a supply of 200 mg ibuprofen and 500 mg acetaminophen at home, you will also want to pick these up prior to your appointment.

How to Eat and How to Dine

After each of my gum grafts, I felt, ate, and slept incredibly well.

The evening following the first graft, the Free Gingival Graft, I merely thinned some plain Greek yogurt with a little milk and called it dinner.

As I mentioned previously, it is normal to experience a little "tinting," as the dental community likes to refer to it, the day of a gum graft procedure. So unless you are eating strawberry or cherry flavored yogurt, you may want to avoid looking too closely at your glass as you drink your first dinner. Just a little heads-up from someone who's already been there.

At bedtime, I crawled in and slept sound as a kitten.

After the second graft, the Soft Tissue Allograft, I thinned some cold Asparagus and Green Pea Vichyssoise with a little milk for my dinner.

Every morning the first few days after each of my gum grafts, breakfast consisted of a sizeable portion of banana and yogurt smoothie followed by as much pre-brewed, sweetened, cold coffee as I wanted. Lunches were more thinned Greek yogurt. And in the evenings, I dined on nutritious chilled soup and a small glass of white wine.

11

" There is absolutely no reason

why you should go around hungry. "

Your Gum Graft Experience

In my case, the recovery period following the gum graft procedures was surprisingly easy, however, the specifics in your case, and even your attitude, may result in a different experience.

Although the weeks following a gum graft are on occasion referred to as "the gum graft diet," there is absolutely no reason why you should go around hungry. In the following section, you will find a variety of healthy recipes that will ensure that you do not feel deprived or bored with your food and that no one will have to prepare two separate meals—one meal for the patient and one meal for everyone else.

By the way, a few months after my second gum graft, I went back for another Allograft procedure. It was the easiest of all. My periodontist first considered an alternative type of graft—a Connective-Tissue Graft, in which tissue would have been taken from underneath a flap of skin at the roof of my mouth—but she determined that I was not a good candidate for that option.

Now that I've had three grafts, I can honestly say it is nothing to be dreaded, delayed, or dodged.

Despite a few stitches, and perhaps a sensitive palate, if you consider the suggestions I have included in this book, as well as closely follow your periodontist's instructions, you too should have a positive gum graft experience. Eat well. Sleep well. And you should be just fine.

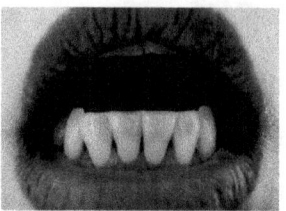

Ready for photos!

〰〰〰〰〰〰〰〰〰〰〰〰〰〰〰〰〰〰〰〰〰〰〰〰〰〰〰〰〰〰〰〰〰〰〰〰

" It's really much easier than you think! "

If you would like some additional tips that I decided were a bit too contentious to include in this book, visit my blog at http://www.susangclark.com.

7 Healthy Recipes

These are the recipes that got me through the first few weeks after my gum grafts.

The fruit and yogurt smoothies are delicious and filling. I suggest that you select fruit that does not have a lot of small seeds that might irritate a tender mouth. I also suggest Greek-style yogurt; it provides twice the protein as some other yogurt.

All the soups can be served pureed and chilled on the first few days following your gum graft, when cold food and liquids are recommended. You may need to thin them with a little milk or broth on the early days. On later days, you can serve the soups warm. If you are cooking for other than yourself or the patient, you can divide the prepared soup and serve half chilled and pureed; serve the other half warm and chunky.

I realize that everyone is not totally at ease in the kitchen, so I've rewritten these recipes for someone with my significant other's level of cooking knowledge. The recipes are very forgiving. The biggest thing that can go wrong is using too high a heat setting. Using a lower heat setting for longer is better.

If you don't cook, look for healthy soups at your supermarket salad bar that can be pureed and chilled at home.

15

" ... these smoothie recipes **do not include ice**, which would dilute the nutritional value and change the consistency of the smoothie prepared for future days. "

FRUIT SMOOTHIES

If you are a fan of unflavored plain yogurt, I recommend Greek-style low-fat or non-fat yogurt. Plain yogurt pairs well with the natural sweetness of ripe fruit. However, if you prefer more sweetness, choose vanilla-flavored yogurt instead. I recommend fresh fruits such as ripe bananas, peaches, or mangoes. Bananas are available year round, relatively inexpensive, and easy to peel, as well as high in fiber, B vitamins, and potassium. A little orange juice preserves the color and allows you to enjoy the smoothie, stored in an airtight pitcher in your refrigerator, for up to three days. Please note that these smoothie recipes **do not include ice**, which would dilute the nutritional value and change the consistency of the smoothie prepared for future days.

One Serving:

1 cup yogurt
1 cup fresh or frozen fruit (bananas, peaches, or mangoes)
splash of orange juice

Two Servings:

2 cups yogurt
2 cups fresh or frozen fruit (bananas, peaches, or mangoes)
¼ cup orange juice

Four Servings:

4 cups yogurt
4 cups fresh ripe or frozen fruit (bananas, peaches, or mangoes)
½ cup orange juice

If you are using fresh fruit, peel and cut it into 1-inch chunks. Frozen fruit should be partially thawed and also be in approximately 1-inch chunks. Place fruit in a pitcher blender. Add orange juice and yogurt. Put lid on blender. Pulse to break up the fruit, then puree the mixture. Refrigerate smoothie in a separate, sealed container.

GREEN PEA SOUP

This soup is quick and simple to prepare. It is mild and easy to swallow on the first or second evening after your procedure. The yogurt gives it stick-to-your-ribs protein. Prepare it ahead of time so that the soup can chill in the refrigerator before time to eat. If you will be drinking your dinner from a wine glass, as I previously suggested, you may need to thin the finished soup with a little milk.

Ingredients:
1 tablespoon butter
1 shallot, peeled and minced
4 cups water
6 cups frozen green peas
¼ teaspoon dried thyme or tarragon
1 cup low-fat or non-fat unflavored plain yogurt
1/8 teaspoon black pepper
salt (optional)

Heat a saucepan on low heat; add butter. Add shallot, sauté 2 minutes. Add water, peas and thyme or tarragon. Raise heat to medium and bring to a low boil. Then reduce heat to low, cover, and cook about 15 minutes, until peas are just tender.

Puree soup with an immersion blender in the pot, or cool slightly and puree in a pitcher blender.

Mix a little soup into yogurt, then stir yogurt and black pepper into soup. Taste. If desired, add 1/8 teaspoon salt. Refrigerate. Serve cold on the first day; serve warm on later days.

" . . . intended to be served chilled,

but it is also delicious warm. "

ASPARAGUS VICHYSSOISE

This soup is intended to be served chilled, but it is also delicious warm. If asparagus is available at an exceptional price, feel free to substitute more asparagus for the green peas. Otherwise, the green peas give the soup a nice bright color while still allowing the asparagus to be the primary flavor.

Ingredients:
1 tablespoon butter
½ sweet onion, diced
1 clove garlic, peeled and minced
1/8 teaspoon dried hot red pepper flakes (optional)
3 ½ cups low-sodium chicken broth
2 medium white potatoes, peeled and diced
¼ teaspoon grated or ground nutmeg
¼ teaspoon ground coriander
¼ teaspoon ground black pepper
1 pound of asparagus, washed, trimmed, and cut in 1-inch pieces
½ cup frozen green peas
1 ½ cups of low-fat or non-fat unflavored plain yogurt
salt (optional)

Heat a large pot on low heat; add butter. After 30 seconds, add onion and cook, stirring occasionally, 5 minutes or until soft. Add garlic and hot red pepper flakes; cook 2 minutes. Add the broth and potatoes, nutmeg, coriander, and black pepper. Raise heat to medium and bring to a low boil. Then reduce heat to low and simmer, uncovered, stirring occasionally, until potatoes are tender.

Add asparagus and green peas and simmer, with lid on, stirring occasionally, until asparagus is fork tender.

Puree with an immersion blender in the pot, or chill slightly and puree in a pitcher blender.

Mix a little soup into yogurt, then stir yogurt mixture into soup. Taste. If desired, add 1/8 teaspoon salt. Serve chilled or warmed.

SAVORY PUMPKIN SOUP

This makes a savory (not sweet) soup. Pumpkin is loaded with antioxidants, vitamins, fiber, and potassium. Yogurt adds protein.

Ingredients:
1 tablespoon olive oil
1 small onion, diced, ¼ inch
1 teaspoon garlic, peeled and minced
1 teaspoon curry powder
1 teaspoon cumin
¼ teaspoon cardamom
¼ teaspoon black pepper
2 cups low-sodium fat-free chicken broth or vegetable broth
1 can plain pumpkin puree (not pumpkin pie filling)
1 ½ cups of low-fat or non-fat unflavored plain yogurt
salt (optional)

Heat a large pot on low heat; add oil. After 30 seconds, add onion and cook 5 minutes or until soft. Add garlic and cook 2 minutes. Add curry, cumin, cardamom, and black pepper. Cook 1 minute, stirring.

Stir in broth and pumpkin. Raise heat to medium and bring to a low boil. Reduce heat to low and simmer for about 20 minutes, stirring occasionally.

Puree all, or half, or none at all. Use an immersion blender in the pot, or chill slightly and puree in a pitcher blender.

Mix a little soup into yogurt, then stir yogurt into soup. Taste. If desired, add 1/8 teaspoon salt. Serve chilled or warmed.

" . . . seasoned with a small amount of Dry Sherry wine

and Sherry vinegar. Be sure to use **both**! "

BLACK BEAN SOUP

This thick, hearty soup is seasoned with a small amount of Dry Sherry wine **and** Sherry vinegar. Be sure to use **both**! It also includes nutrition-rich pumpkin. For a vegetarian soup, omit the ham and use vegetable broth.

Ingredients:
1 tablespoon of butter or olive oil
2 cups of onion, diced
3 garlic cloves, peeled and minced
2 tablespoons ground cumin
1/8 teaspoon cayenne pepper (¼ teaspoon, if you like more heat)
4 cans of black beans, rinsed and drained, or a 1 pound dried black beans, cooked and drained
4 cups low-salt beef, chicken, or vegetable broth
1 can plain pumpkin puree (not pumpkin pie filling)
½ teaspoon black pepper
2 14 oz. cans of diced tomatoes
1/3 cup Dry Sherry wine
3 to 4 Tablespoons Sherry vinegar
¼ pound low-salt cooked deli ham, cut into 1/4-inch dice (optional)
salt (optional)

Heat a large pot on low heat; add butter or oil. Add onion and cook 5 minutes or until soft. Add garlic and cook 2 minutes. Add cumin and cayenne pepper and cook 1 minute, stirring.

Stir in black beans, broth, pumpkin, black pepper, and tomatoes. Stir in the Dry Sherry wine. Raise heat to medium and bring to a low boil. Then reduce to low heat and simmer about 25 minutes, with lid on, stirring occasionally.

Puree all, or half, or none at all. Use an immersion blender in the pot, or chill slightly and puree in a pitcher blender.

Just before serving, add Sherry vinegar and, if using, the diced ham. Taste. If desired, add 1/8 teaspoon salt. Serve chilled or warmed.

CHICKPEA AND SPINACH SOUP

I have heard that peanuts were brought to America from Africa, where they were often ground into a paste to thicken and flavor soups and stews, as well as increase protein. For vegetarian soup, omit the chicken and reduce the vegetable broth total to 3 cups.

Ingredients:
2 teaspoons olive oil
1 medium onion, diced, ¼ inch (about 1 cup)
1 pound of chicken breast, cut into ½-inch pieces
1 clove garlic, peeled and minced, 1/8 inch (about 1 teaspoon)
1 teaspoon paprika
1 teaspoon ground coriander
1/8 teaspoon cayenne pepper (¼ teaspoon, if you like more heat)
¼ cup smooth peanut butter
4 cups low-sodium chicken broth or vegetable broth (divided)
1 can chickpeas, rinsed and drained
1 small sweet potato, peeled and diced, ¼ inch
1 small red bell pepper, diced, ¼ inch
1 can diced tomatoes
2 cups chopped spinach, fresh or frozen
¼ teaspoon black pepper
salt (optional)

Either cook the chicken breasts whole on an aluminum foil-covered shallow pan in a 400-degree oven or toaster oven for 15 to 20 minutes, cool slightly and cut into ½-inch pieces OR cut up the raw chicken and cook it in the oil and onions before adding the garlic.

27

Heat a large pot on low heat; add oil. After 30 seconds, add onion and cook 5 minutes or until soft. Add garlic and cook 2 minutes. Add paprika, coriander, and cayenne to onion mixture. Cook 1 minute, stirring.

In a measuring cup mix the peanut butter with ½ cup of broth to make a smooth paste.

Add the peanut butter mixture, the remaining broth, chickpeas, sweet potato, red bell pepper, tomatoes, and cooked chicken to the pot. Stir. Raise temperature to medium and bring to a low boil. Reduce the heat to low and, with lid on, simmer, stirring often, until sweet potato is fork tender. Stir in spinach and cook until the spinach is just wilted. Add black pepper.

Puree all, or half, or none at all. Use an immersion blender in the pot, or chill slightly and puree in a pitcher blender.

Taste. If desired, add 1/8 teaspoon salt. Serve chilled or warmed.

SPICY VEGETARIAN SOUP

While this version of an African-inspired soup is very satisfying, it requires fewer ingredients so it is quicker to make and is more economical. Peanut butter and plain yogurt provide protein. This recipe serves three, so double the recipe if more is needed. Note: The heat from the fresh ginger may not be appreciated by young children.

Ingredients:
1 tablespoon olive oil
1 yellow onion, chopped (about 1 cup)
1 medium carrot, peeled and finely chopped (about 3/4 cup)
1 to 2 teaspoons peeled, minced fresh ginger (kicks up the heat!)
½ teaspoon coriander
½ teaspoon paprika
1 sweet potato, peeled and chopped (about 1 cup)
2 cups of low-sodium chicken broth or vegetable broth
½ cup tomato juice or ½ cup water and 1 teaspoon tomato paste
¼ teaspoon ground black pepper
¼ - ½ cup creamy peanut butter
¾ cup of low-fat or non-fat unflavored plain yogurt
salt (optional)

Heat a large saucepan on low heat; add olive oil. After 30 seconds, add onion and carrots and cook 5 minutes, stirring often, or until soft. Add ginger and cook 2 minutes. Add paprika and coriander to onion mixture. Cook 1 minute, stirring.

Add sweet potato, broth, black pepper, and tomato juice. Raise heat to medium and bring mixture to a low boil, then reduce to low heat and, with lid on, simmer about 15 minutes, stirring often, until the sweet potatoes are fork tender.

Stir in the peanut butter. Puree soup with an immersion blender, or cool slightly and puree in a pitcher blender.

Mix a little soup into yogurt, then stir yogurt mixture into soup. Taste. If desired, add 1/8 teaspoon salt. Serve chilled or warmed.

Connect with Susan

I really hope that you enjoyed this book and that it helped you to become more comfortable with what to expect and what you can do to make the first few days following your gum graft as easy as possible.

As a self-published author, my reviews come directly from my readers. I would so appreciate it if you would leave a review for this book. A single sentence, or even a kind word, would mean so much, and it would help this book get found by others who might also benefit from it. Please leave your review on the book's Amazon page at http://www.amazon.com/author/susangclark.

If you have any questions or just want to connect, I'd love to hear from you.

My website is http://www.susangclark.com
My email address is Susan@susangclark.com
On Twitter, https://twitter.com/SusanGClark
On Pinterest, http://www.pinterest.com/susangclark
On Facebook, https://www.facebook.com/SusanGClarkAuthor

Sincerely,

Susan

PS: Subscribe to Susan's e-mail at http://www.susangclark.com to receive her free assessment for determining if you are stuck in humdrum plus tips to help you transition from humdrum to holy crap! You will also receive occasional notices about new blog posts, books, and instructional videos.

" I'd love to hear from you. "

About the Author

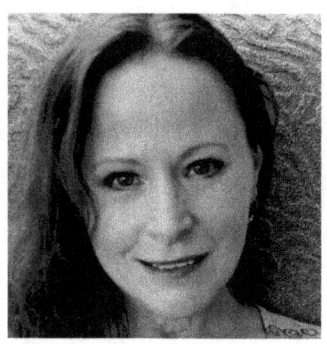

SUSAN G. CLARK is the author of the book *Your Gum Graft: What to Expect & How to Make it Easy! (Including 7 Healthy Recipes)*, as well as the forthcoming book *Swanky Yoga Ropes Wall: How to Build Yours and Enjoy A Healthy Back, Stable Weight & Balanced Life*. Following will be the first in her book series on honoring your holy crap! moments.

Susan is dedicated to inspiring people to transition from humdrum to holy crap! through her mostly true, often embarrassingly personal essays, which have appeared in the magazines Pets, Sasee, and The Quilt Life, and through her blog at http://www.susangclark.com/blog.

Her early career included stints as a marketing copy editor, a page designer, an academic journal assistant editor, and an events planner. Interspersed throughout those pursuits, Susan followed her muse into women's millinery, fine art sales, and jazz radio announcing. Currently, in her downtime she creates fabric collage art for an upcoming children's book and treats herself to a daily yoga practice.

Susan lives in Raleigh, North Carolina, with an almost perfect guy, two rollicking overgrown kittens, and an imaginary dog.

She welcomes your inquiries!

Susan@susangclark.com